THE SWEET ESCAPE GUIDE FOR BEGINNERS

Unleash Your Sweet Freedom, Transform Your Relationship with Sugar, and Ignite a Healthier You

A 3-Week Challenge for Doubtful First-Timers

Dr Alton

THE SWEET ESCAPE GUIDE FOR BEGINNERS

Copyright © [2024] by Dr Alton

Protected by copyright law. No piece of this distribution might be imitated, disseminated, or communicated in any structure or using any and all means, including copying, recording, or other electronic or mechanical techniques, without the earlier composed authorization of the distributer, with the exception of brief citations epitomized in basic surveys and certain other noncommercial purposes allowed by intellectual property regulation.

Table of Contents

Contents

**THE SWEET ESCAPE GUIDE FOR
BEGINNERS**

THE SWEET ESCAPE GUIDE FOR BEGINNERS

**THE SWEET ESCAPE GUIDE FOR
BEGINNERS**

Introduction

Leaving on an excursion to break liberated from the shackles of sugar could appear to be overwhelming, particularly for the people who are wary or new to the idea. In any case, dread not, for "The Sweet Departure Guide for Fledglings" is here to direct you through an extraordinary 3-week challenge that will rethink your relationship with sugar and prepare to a better, more dynamic you.

Week 1: Breaking the Chains

In the initial week, we jump profound into figuring out your ongoing relationship with sugar. We'll assist you with distinguishing those tricky secret sugars hiding in your kitchen and guide you through a groundbreaking kitchen detox. It is time to welcome healthier alternatives and say goodbye to sugary culprits. This week sets the stage, permitting you to lay out reasonable objectives and venture out towards sweet opportunity.

Week 2: The Secret Remedy for Cravings

Week 2 is devoted to revealing the secret remedy, as cravings frequently bind us to the sugar cycle. Learn the science behind cravings and how to tell the difference between physical and mental triggers. Figure out how to end the propensity circle and fulfill your sweet tooth normally. Savvy nibbling, careful eating practices, and understanding the brain science behind desires will engage you to vanquish these apparently unfavorable obstacles.

Week 3: Adoring Food Without Sugar

As the test advances, Week 3 welcomes you to experience passionate feelings for food once more, without the prop of sugar. Find the lavishness of flavors in entire food sources, investigating the culinary world with spices and flavors. This week is all about embracing the joy of cooking and developing a long-term relationship with food through intuitive eating. Celebrate little triumphs as you reclassify enjoying a delightful, satisfying feast.

Examples of overcoming adversity and Tributes

Interlaced all through the aide are rousing examples of overcoming adversity and ardent tributes from those who've gone through this sweet break venture. Understand that you are in good company as you continued looking for sweet opportunity, and witness the significant effect this challenge has had on the prosperity of others.

Conclusion: Embrace Your Sweet Opportunity

As the 3-week challenge comes to a nearby, pause for a minute to consider your excursion. Feel empowered after releasing yourself from sugar's grip. This is much more than a guide; It is the road map that will lead you to sweet freedom and a happier, healthier you. Touch off the flash inside and relish the sweet taste of progress as you step into a future where you are in charge, and sugar is presently not the expert of your wellbeing. Welcome to "The Sweet Departure Guide for Amateurs" - your vital aspect for releasing sweet opportunity and changing your life.

THE SWEET ESCAPE GUIDE FOR BEGINNERS

Forward

1.1 Why Sugar Detox?

Setting out on a sugar detox isn't simply a momentary wellbeing pattern yet a cognizant choice to recover command over your prosperity. In a world immersed with sweet enticements, understanding the need for a sugar detox is vital. Unreasonable sugar utilization has been connected to a heap of medical problems, including heftiness, diabetes, and cardiovascular illnesses. Sugar can harm energy levels, mood stability, and cognitive function in addition to its physical effects. A sugar detox fills in as a reset button for your body, permitting you to break

THE SWEET ESCAPE GUIDE FOR BEGINNERS

liberated from the habit-forming cycle and prepare for a better, more empowered life.

1.2 Advantages of a Sugar Detox

The advantages of a sugar detox reach out a long ways past simple weight the board. This excursion holds the commitment of significant changes for both your physical and mental prosperity. By dispensing with or essentially decreasing sugar admission, you can expect expanded energy levels, further developed concentration, and better rest. Besides, a sugar detox can be an impetus for upgraded mind-set and a more steady profound state. Your taste buds will go through a restoration, turning out to be more receptive to the regular pleasantness of entire food varieties. Also, breaking liberated from sugar's grasp can add to long haul wellbeing, decreasing the gamble of persistent sicknesses and advancing in general essentialness.

1.3 Laying out Reasonable Objectives

Laying out reasonable objectives is the foundation of an effective sugar detox. There's really no need to focus on making radical, unreasonable changes for the time being yet rather taking on a slow, economical methodology. Set objectives that are in line with your preferences and lifestyle, taking into account your current relationship with sugar. Whether it's decreasing everyday sugar consumption, distinguishing and wiping out secret sugars, or continuously changing to better other options, your objectives ought to be explicit, quantifiable, and reachable. Setting little achievements en route permits you to follow progress and celebrate triumphs, cultivating a positive outlook all through the detox venture. Keep in mind, the key is to make a guide that engages you to explore the difficulties of sugar detox while building an establishment for dependable wellbeing and prosperity.

2. Figuring out Sugar

Sugar, an omnipresent piece of present day eats less, assumes a huge part in our general wellbeing. Understanding the subtleties of sugar is critical for pursuing informed decisions about what we consume. This part dives into the sorts of sugar, their sources, and the effect they have on our prosperity.

2.1 Kinds of Sugar

2.1.1 Normal versus Added Sugars

Separating among normal and added sugars is the most vital phase in fathoming the sugar scene. Regular sugars happen naturally in food sources like natural products (fructose) and dairy items (lactose). These sugars come packaged with fundamental supplements and fiber, moderating their effect on glucose levels. Then again, added sugars are those integrated into handled food varieties and drinks during assembling. The test lies in recognizing and limiting added sugar utilization, as it frequently adds to exorbitant caloric admission absent any and all dietary advantages.

2.1.2 Secret Sugars in Food varieties

Exploring the basic food item path can be precarious because of the presence of stowed away sugars in apparently guiltless items. This subsection uncovers the secret wellsprings of sugar, uncovering terms like high-fructose corn syrup, maltose, or even dissipated stick juice. Attention to these nom de plumes enables people to settle on additional cognizant decisions and pick entire, natural food sources.

2.2 Effect of Sugar on Wellbeing

Sugar's effect stretches out past simple pleasantness; it altogether impacts our wellbeing. The effects of eating too much sugar are numerous, ranging from contributing to obesity and weight gain to raising the risk of type 2 diabetes and heart disease. Diving into the physiological impacts of sugar gives a more clear comprehension of why control is vital.

2.3 Suggested Everyday Recompense

Laying out a suggested everyday recompense (RDA) for sugar consumption helps with making benchmarks for a decent eating regimen. Rules set by wellbeing associations offer experiences into the ideal amount of sugar utilization to keep up with in general wellbeing. Perceiving these proposals permits people to settle on cognizant conclusions about their everyday sugar consumption, cultivating a way of life lined up with long haul prosperity.

Individuals are equipped with the knowledge necessary to make healthier dietary choices when they are aware of the intricate nature of sugar. By knowing among regular and added sugars, recognizing stowed away sources, getting a handle on the wellbeing suggestions, and sticking to suggested everyday recompenses, one can leave on a way towards a more careful and adjusted way to deal with sugar utilization.

3. Getting ready for Your Detox

Setting out on a sugar detox requires key preparation and a careful way to deal with your current circumstance and dietary decisions. This part frames the fundamental stages for setting up your kitchen and feasts to make way for a fruitful detox venture.

3.1 Kitchen Makeover

3.1.1 Recognizing and Eliminating Sweet Food varieties

The most important phase in planning for your detox is leading a careful assessment of your kitchen.

Distinguish and eliminate any sweet guilty parties concealing in your storage space, cooler, or ledges. This incorporates things with added sugars, sweet tidbits, and handled food sources that add to unnecessary sugar admission. Getting your space free from these enticements is a critical push toward establishing a strong climate for your sugar detox.

3.1.2 Loading up on Solid Other options

With the old clearing a path for the new, stock your kitchen with different healthy other options. Supplant sweet snacks with supplement rich choices like new organic products, nuts, and seeds. Decide on entire grains, lean proteins, and a vivid exhibit of vegetables to frame the groundwork of your feasts. A well-stocked kitchen not only ensures that you will have access to healthier options, but it will also make the switch to a sugar-free lifestyle more enjoyable.

3.2 Dinner Arranging

3.2.1 Adjusted Dinners

Dinner arranging is a foundation of a fruitful sugar detox. Configuration adjusted dinners that incorporate a blend of lean proteins, complex carbs, and sound fats. Consolidate a rainbow of vegetables to boost healthful variety. Make progress toward dinners that satisfy your appetite as well as give supported energy over the course of the day. Adjusting macronutrients guarantees you get the vital supplements without depending on sugar-loaded choices.

3.2.2 Nibble Choices

Nibbling can be an expected entanglement during a sugar detox, however it doesn't need to be. Prepare for fulfilling and nutritious bites that line up with your objectives. New organic product, Greek yogurt, vegetable sticks with hummus, and a small bunch of nuts are great decisions. Having these options promptly accessible limits the compulsion to go after sweet tidbits when appetite strikes between dinners.

Setting up your kitchen and dinners is a proactive and enabling move toward a fruitful sugar detox. You are creating an environment that supports your journey to sweet freedom by identifying and eliminating sugary foods, stocking up on healthier alternatives, and planning well-balanced meals and snacks. The cautious curtain of your kitchen establishes the vibe for the weeks ahead, guaranteeing a smooth and charming progress to a without sugar way of life.

4. Sugar Detox Diet

Setting out on a sugar detox includes a conscious shift towards an eating routine that focuses on entire, supplement thick food varieties while limiting or killing added sugars. This part gives a manual for embracing a sugar detox diet, underlining an entire food sources approach and offering test dinner plans for different times.

4.1 Entire Food sources Approach

A foundation of the sugar detox diet is the entire food sources approach. Embrace various entire, natural food sources to guarantee you get fundamental supplements without the secret sugars tracked down in many handled choices. Load your plate with brilliant vegetables, lean proteins, entire grains, and solid fats. Entire food varieties support your healthful requirements as well as add to a more maintained and adjusted energy over the course of the day.

4.2 Sample Meal Plans

4.2.1 Ideas for Breakfast Greek Yogurt Parfait:

Greek yogurt with no additional sugars

Blended berries

Almonds or chia seeds for crunch

Vegetable Omelet:

Eggs with sautéed spinach, tomatoes, and ringer peppers

Avocado cuts as an afterthought

4.2.2 Lunch and Supper Recipes

Barbecued Chicken Serving of mixed greens:

Barbecued chicken bosom on a bed of leafy greens

Cherry tomatoes, cucumber, and feta cheddar

Olive oil and balsamic vinegar dressing

Quinoa Pan fried food:

Quinoa sautéed with different brilliant vegetables

Tofu or lean protein of decision

Soy sauce and ginger for some zing

Prepared Salmon with Yam Pound:

Prepared salmon filet

Crushed yams prepared with a sprinkle of cinnamon

4.2.3 Nibble Ideas

Apple Cuts with Almond Spread:

Fresh apple cuts with a tablespoon of almond margarine

Vegetable Sticks with Hummus:

Carrot, cucumber, and ringer pepper sticks with hummus

4.3 Hydration Tips

Remaining enough hydrated is a critical part of any detox venture. Decide on water as your essential refreshment, holding back nothing eight glasses per day. Home grown teas and injected water with cuts of lemon, cucumber, or mint can change it up without the requirement for added sugars. Limit or kill sweet beverages, including soft drinks and certain natural product juices, to keep up with the virtue of your sugar detox.

This sugar detox diet not only helps people have a better relationship with food, but it also helps them stay energetic and feel good in general. By embracing entire food sources and integrating these example dinner thoughts into your daily practice, you're establishing the groundwork for an effective and charming sugar detox venture.

5. Exploring Desires

Desires can be imposing foes during a sugar detox, however understanding and addressing them head-on is vital to a fruitful excursion. This segment investigates the brain research behind sugar desires, gives choices to fulfill your sweet tooth strongly, and energizes the act of careful eating.

5.1 Figuring out Sugar Desires

Unwinding the secret of sugar desires is fundamental for beating them. Frequently, desires are about the body's requirement for pleasantness as well as can be connected to close to home triggers, stress, or propensity. Perceiving the contrast among physical and profound desires enables you to properly answer. Keeping a diary to recognize examples and triggers is an important device in grasping your desires.

5.2 Sound Choices to Fulfill Sweet Tooth

Hankering something sweet doesn't mean surrendering to refined sugars. All things being equal, investigate a collection of solid options that fulfill your sweet tooth as well as add to your general prosperity. Settle on:

New Natural product:

Natural candy with a lot of fiber and sugar from nature.

Berries, mangoes, and apples are superb decisions.

Dim Chocolate:

Pick top notch dull chocolate with a cocoa content of 70% or higher.

A little piece can give a wonderful sweet fix.

Date Energy Chomps:

Mix dates, nuts, and a touch of cinnamon for a normally sweet and energy-supporting tidbit.

Parfait de yogurt:

Greek yogurt with a shower of honey and a sprinkle of nuts or granola.

5.3 Careful Eating Practices

Careful eating is an amazing asset to explore desires and develop a better relationship with food.

Integrate the accompanying practices into your daily schedule:

Enjoy Each Chomp:

Take your time eating and enjoy the flavors of your food.

Take note of the chewing motion, aromas, and textures.

Pay attention to Appetite Signs:

Check out your body's appetite and completion signals.

Eat when you're eager and stop when you're fulfilled.

Take out Interruptions:

Limit interruptions during feasts, like screens or performing various tasks.

Center around the demonstration of eating and the joy it brings.

Practice Appreciation:

Prior to eating, pause for a minute to offer thanks for your food.

Develop a positive and mindful approach to food preparation.

By figuring out the foundations of sugar desires, consolidating sound other options, and rehearsing careful eating, you not just explore the difficulties of a sugar detox all the more successfully yet in addition encourage a more profound association with the food you eat. With this mindful approach, cravings become opportunities to build a healthier relationship with your body and the nourishment it deserves rather than obstacles.

6. Remaining Dynamic

Active work is a fundamental part of an all encompassing way to deal with wellbeing, supplementing the advantages of a sugar detox. In this segment, we investigate the advantageous connection among exercise and detoxification, as well as give proposals to exercises that line up with your detox process.

6.1 Activity and Detox

Taking part in standard activity isn't just valuable for generally wellbeing yet in addition assumes a strong part in the detoxification cycle. Actual work animates blood course, speeds up the lymphatic framework, and improves the proficiency of the body's normal detox instruments. Whether it's through perspiring, further developed processing, or expanded oxygenation of tissues, practice adds to the end of poisons and supports the body's capacity to adjust to a without sugar way of life.

6.2 Suggested Exercises

Integrating various exercises into your routine guarantees a balanced way to deal with remaining dynamic during your sugar detox.

Think about the accompanying suggestions:

Cardiovascular Activity:

Energetic Strolling: An open and viable type of activity.

Running or Running: Supports digestion and deliveries endorphins.

Cycling: Fun and low-impact for people of all fitness levels.

Strength Preparing:

Exercises with your own body weight: Squats, lurches, and push-ups further develop muscle tone.

Opposition Preparing: Integrate loads or opposition groups for added challenge.

Mind-Body Practices:

Yoga: Upgrades adaptability, equilibrium, and care.

Pilates: focuses on core strength and flexibility as a whole.

Judo or Qigong: Advances unwinding and careful development.

Stop and go aerobic exercise (HIIT):

Short Eruptions of Extraordinary Activity: Productive for consuming calories and working on cardiovascular wellbeing.

Include Bodyweight Exercises: Hopping jacks, burgees, and hikers.

Outside Exercises:

Hiking: A reviving method for interfacing with nature and remain dynamic.

Swimming: Gives a full-body exercise and is kind with the joints.

High-intensity exercise in a Recreation area: Use seats and open spaces for a different exercise.

Keep in mind, the key is to pick exercises that you appreciate to keep up with consistency. Go for the gold 150 minutes of moderate-power practice each week, or 75 minutes of overwhelming force work out, notwithstanding strength preparing no less than two times every week. Remaining dynamic upgrades the detox interaction as well as adds to generally speaking prosperity, supporting your excursion towards a better, more stimulated way of life.

7. Following Progression

As you leave on your sugar detox adventure, noticing your progression is major for staying roused and keeping an inspirational perspective. The most effective ways to monitor your physical and mental advancement and to commend accomplishments are framed in this part.

7.1 Journaling Keeping

A devoted diary can be a valuable instrument for monitoring your advancement through the sugar detox. Step by step instructions to capitalize on it:

Ordinary Food Log: Report your meals, goodies, and beverages, zeroing in on sugar content. Ponder how your body answers different food choices.

Profound Appraisals: Monitor your day's temperament and energy levels. Perceiving plans among sentiments and wants gives critical encounters.

Craving Diary: Record events of sugar wants, their triggers, and the strategies you use to beat them. This guides in the distinguishing proof of examples and the making of effective ways of dealing with stress.

Dynamic work Tracker: Monitor your day to day work-out schedules, including the sort, term, and power of every action. This strengthens the connection between actual employment and prosperity.

Reflections: Every day, take a moment to reflect on your accomplishments, challenges, and any acquired knowledge. Put forth objectives and recognize your endeavors for the next day.

7.2 Physical and Profound prosperity Enrollments

Common enrollments with both your physical and mental success are indispensable pieces of following your sugar detox progress.

Actual assessments:

Biometric Examinations: Screen changes in weight, body assessments, and, surprisingly, circulatory strain if material.

Energy Levels: Look at your general degree of energy. Could it be that you are experiencing fewer energy crashes throughout the day?

Profound health Enlistments:

Levels of Temperament and Stress: Ponder your personality and sensations of uneasiness. Observe any changes in flexibility to stress and dependability of temperament.

Mental Capacity: Notice overhauls in fixation, center, and mental clarity.

7.3 Noticing Accomplishments

Praising accomplishments, paying little heed to how little, is critical for staying aware of motivation and developing specific inclinations.

Step by step Achievements: Acclaim the completing of each and every week without added sugars. Perceive the work you've done and the positive changes you've seen.

Weight decrease or Body Changes: If losing weight is a goal, congratulations should be given for specific accomplishments. Revolve around non-scale wins like extended muscle tone or further developed health levels.

Chipped away at Thriving: Celebrate updates in energy levels, better rest, and an in everyday superior sensation of flourishing.

Care for Yourself: Plan little, irrelevant compensations for huge achievements. This could consolidate a spa day, another book, or an entertainment development you appreciate.

By merging journaling, conventional prosperity enlistments, and lauding accomplishments, you gain huge encounters into your headway as well as foster a positive and empowering mindset all through your sugar detox adventure. Following your achievements gives unquestionable evidence of your undertakings and desires continued with obligation to a superior lifestyle.

8. Social Support

Going on a sugar detox can be an exciting adventure, and having a strong network of emotionally supportive people is essential to progress. This part examines the meaning of social help and proposes ways of interfacing with individuals who can assist you with detoxing from sugar.

8.1 Maintaining Open and Clear Communication with Family and Friends

During your sugar detox, it is essential to maintain open and clear communication with family and friends. Share your targets, clarifications behind attempt the detox, and the assist you with truly caring about. This is how to improve comprehension:

Show Loved ones: Help your friends and family with understanding the reasons for your sugar detox and the beneficial outcome it can have on your prosperity.

Request Joint effort: Demand their assistance in laying out a without sugar environment at home. Encourage better food choices at communal feasts.

Plan trips with companions: Give thoughts for social exercises that don't fixate on food or better other

THE SWEET ESCAPE GUIDE FOR BEGINNERS

options. This can consolidate outdoors works out, wellbeing classes, or regardless, cooking alongside sans sugar recipes.

Express Cutoff points: Clearly bestow your cutoff points regarding allurements or strain to gobble up sweet food sources. A solid circle will respect your decisions.

8.2 Joining Sugar Detox Social class

Communicating with comparative individuals who are on a tantamount outing can give a sensation of neighborhood, experiences, and significant clues. Contemplate the going with:

Online Social class: Join sugar detox bundles through electronic amusement stages or conversations where people share pieces of information, troubles, and instances of beating affliction.

Close by Care Gatherings: Investigate health focuses or local gatherings in your space that host sugar detox-related occasions and gatherings. Especially strong associations can be made face to face.

Companions of Responsibility: Working together with someone who has similar goals makes a genuinely steady organization where you can convince each other and share the ups and downs of the detox cycle.

8.3 Searching for Capable Course

Occasionally, searching for capable course can offer redid help and expertise. Contemplate the accompanying choices:

Nutritionist or Dietitian: Chat with a food master to make a tweaked sugar detox plan specially designed to your dietary tendencies and prosperity needs.

Expert or Mentor: If up close and personal eating or more significant mental factors are involved, searching for the heading of a subject matter expert or educator can give critical pieces of information and strategy for practical adaptations.

Mentor in Wellness: Working with a wellness expert can assist you with making an activity plan that accommodates your sugar detox goals and works on your general wellbeing.

Remember that each individual's way to a sans sugar way of life is novel. An extensive emotional support network is formed by forming a strong group of friends, family, and like-minded individuals and seeking expert guidance when necessary. The likelihood of successfully navigating the challenges of a sugar detox and embracing a healthier lifestyle is increased when you surround yourself with comfort and understanding.

9. Dealing with Difficulties

Misfortunes are a characteristic piece of any groundbreaking excursion, and a sugar detox is no special case. This part gives direction on recognizing triggers and compelling procedures for recovering energy when confronted with mishaps.

9.1 Recognizing Triggers

Understanding the variables that add to difficulties is a pivotal move toward defeating them. This is the way to recognize and explore triggers:

Stress: High-feelings of anxiety can prompt profound eating and desires for sweet solace food sources. Perceive stressors in your day to day existence and investigate elective survival strategies like contemplation or exercise.

Social Circumstances: Occasions or social events where sweet treats are bountiful may present difficulties. Prepare, bring your own without sugar options, and impart your dietary decisions to everyone around you.

Close to home Triggers: Profound states like bitterness, weariness, or dissatisfaction can set off desires for sweet food varieties. Recognize close to home triggers and foster better ways of adapting, like taking part in a leisure activity or connecting with a companion.

Ecological Signals: Cravings can be sparked by particular routines or environments. Monitoring these signals permits you to proactively change your environmental factors or propensities.

9.2 Methodologies for Refocusing

Misfortunes are not disappointments but rather valuable chances to learn and rearrange. Utilize these methodologies to recover concentration and proceed with your sugar detox venture:

Practice Self-Empathy: Comprehend that misfortunes are a characteristic piece of any change cycle. Accept the setback, be kind to yourself, and let go of any guilt.

Reflect and Learn: Examine the factors that contributed to the setback. What set off the deviation from your arrangement? Use mishaps as growth opportunities to refine your methodology pushing ahead.

Reaffirm Your Objectives: Return to your underlying purposes behind endeavor the sugar detox. Reiterate your commitment to healthier food choices, more energy, and improved health.

Plan for What's in store: Expect possible moves and devise systems to defeat them. Having an arrangement set up prepares you to explore comparable circumstances all the more successfully later on.

Look for Help: Contact your encouraging group of people, whether it's companions, family, or a sugar detox local area. Share your experience, and rest on others for consolation and direction.

Restore Schedule: As soon as possible, return to your regular routine. Consistency is vital to building propensities, and refocusing expeditiously supports your obligation to the detox cycle.

Keep in mind, mishaps are not characteristic of disappointment, yet rather amazing open doors for development and strength. You can improve your capacity to overcome obstacles and continue making progress toward a sugar-free lifestyle by recognizing triggers, gaining knowledge from setbacks, and employing effective strategies.

Certainly! Let's expand on Week 1's material: Breaking the Chains.

Week 1: Breaking the Chains

2.1 Grasping Your Sugar Relationship

2.1.1 Distinguishing Stowed away Sugars

Sugar conceals in startling spots, frequently under names that aren't quickly conspicuous. In this segment, we'll give an exhaustive rundown of elective names for sugar found on food marks. Understanding these monikers is critical for perceiving and keeping away from stowed away sugars in your eating regimen.

2.1.2 Surveying Your Ongoing Sugar Admission

Investigate your everyday eating routine. Utilizing a food diary or a sustenance application, track your sugar utilization over a run of the mill week. This mindfulness practice assists you with perceiving designs, distinguish pain points, and sets you up for the impending detox.

2.2 Kitchen Detox

2.2.1 Clearing Sweet Food sources

Change your kitchen into a without sugar zone. Figure out how to recognize and dispose of normal sweet guilty parties sneaking in your storage room and refrigerator. We'll direct you through a bit by bit interaction to clean up your kitchen, making it a steady climate for your sugar detox venture.

2.2.2 Loading up on Healthy Other options

It's not just about what you eliminate; It also depends on what you add. Find a list of healthy substitutes for sugary snacks and ingredients. We'll give a shopping rundown of nutritious staples that will act as the establishment for your better dietary patterns.

2.3 Establishing Achievable

Objectives for the First Week After laying the groundwork, it is time to establish attainable objectives for the first week. These objectives ought to be explicit, quantifiable, and custom-made to your own difficulties and way of life. Whether it's decreasing sugar consumption by a specific rate or attempting another without sugar recipe, these objectives will keep you engaged and inspired all through the underlying period of your sugar detox.

Remember to include practical advice, inspirational quotes, and perhaps even recipes that are appropriate for each section as your guide develops. Along these lines, peruses can apply the information they gain straightforwardly to their regular routines during the sugar detox challenge.

We absolutely need to get into the content for Week 2: The Secret Answer for Wants.

3.1 The Science behind Desires

3.1.1 Actual versus Mental Desires Reveal the two essential sorts of desires: those that are set off by authentic actual necessities and those that are set off by mental elements. The following is the secret treatment for cravings: Understanding the capability draws in you to answer wants all the more effectively. We'll research how to perceive and address each sort to develop a superior relationship with food.

3.1.2 Stopping the Penchant Circle

Wants much of the time become consistent approaches to acting. Track down ways of bringing an end to the propensity circle, which incorporates the sign, the daily schedule, and the award. We'll give you important tips to replace sweet cravings with healthier alternatives, assisting you in making long-lasting dietary changes.

3.2 A Usually Satisfying Sweet Tooth

Find satiating and nutritious bites that won't halt your progress through the sugar detox. We'll guide you through picking snacks affluent in fiber, sound fats, and proteins, keeping you fulfilled and helping with checking sugar wants between meals.

3.2.2 Merging Sweet Flavors in Galas

Explore standard sugars and trimmings that add enjoyableness to your blowouts without the unfavorable outcomes of refined sugars. We'll show you inventive ways of upgrading the kind of your dinners without utilizing added sugars, utilizing anything from organic products to flavors.

3.3 Careful Eating Habits

Develop a careful eating habit that will help you enjoy your meals and better recognize signs of hunger and fullness. We will discuss care strategies that assist individuals with having a superior relationship with food and make it doubtful that they settle on indiscreet and profound food decisions.

All through the ongoing week's substance, embed practical models, individual records, and natural parts that ask perusers to successfully attract with the material. Close to the completion of Week 2, perusers should have a device reserve of methods to manage and overcome sugar wants in a legitimate and enchanting way.

Certainly! How about we investigate the substance for Week 3: Cherishing Food Without Sugar.

Week 3: Adoring Food without Sugar

4.1 Rediscovering Flavor in Entire Food varieties

4.1.1 Cooking with Spices and Flavors

Jump into the universe of spices and flavors to improve the kinds of your dinners. Find out about various spices and flavors that can add profundity and wealth to your dishes, permitting you to appreciate tasty and fulfilling dinners without depending on added sugars.

4.1.2 Investigating New Fixings

Extend your culinary skylines by presenting different new, entire fixings into your feasts. Find the healthful advantages and novel kinds of various natural products, vegetables, grains, and proteins. We'll give straightforward and delectable recipes that integrate these new fixings into your day to day collection.

4.2 Structure an Economical Relationship with Food

4.2.1 Instinctive Eating

Shift your concentration from prohibitive eating to instinctive eating. Comprehend and answer your body's craving and completion prompts, permitting you to appreciate food without responsibility. We'll direct you through the standards of instinctive eating and what it can emphatically mean for your general prosperity.

4.2.2 partaking During the time spent Cooking

Transform dinner planning into a pleasurable and careful experience. Investigate the delight of cooking by exploring different avenues regarding recipes, attempting new strategies, and embracing the innovative part of setting up your feasts. Find out how having a positive relationship with food can make you feel better and make you less likely to want sugary treats.

4.3 Observing Little Triumphs

Recognize and praise the headway you've made all through the 3-week challenge. Consider the positive improves on in your propensities, energy levels, and by and large prosperity. We'll give tips on defining new objectives for proceeded with progress and keeping a sugar-cognizant way of life pushing ahead.

All through Week 3, urge peruses to share their encounters, evaluate new recipes, and praise their accomplishments in a steady local area. Before the week's over, peruses ought to feel enabled to proceed with their excursion of cherishing food without the requirement for overabundance sugar, cultivating a practical and pleasant relationship with their feasts.

Examples of overcoming adversity and Tributes

5.1 Motivating Accounts of Change

5.1.1 [Reader's Name] - From Sugar Dependence on Sweet Opportunity

Share an individual story of a peruse who effectively finished the 3-week sugar detox challenge. Feature their underlying battles, the particular advances they took, and the positive changes they encountered. Include details about how they overcame obstacles and any unanticipated advantages they discovered along the way.

5.1.2 [Reader's Name] - Adopting a Healthier Lifestyle Tell the story of another reader about how the sugar detox affects all aspects of life. Examine enhancements in energy levels, mental clearness, rest quality, and generally temperament. Give subtleties on the peruser's #1 recipes and methodologies that assisted them with supporting a sugar-cognizant way of life.

5.2 The Effect of Sweet Opportunity on Prosperity

5.2.1 Actual Prosperity

Investigate what lessening sugar consumption emphatically means for actual wellbeing. Remember bits of knowledge from wellbeing specialists for themes, for example, weight the board, further developed glucose levels, and improved cardiovascular wellbeing. Delineate the association between a diminished sugar diet and expanded energy levels.

5.2.2 Mental and Emotional Health

Talk about how sugar consumption affects mental health. Share tributes from perusers who experienced upgrades in state of mind, diminished uneasiness, and expanded mental lucidity subsequent to finishing the sugar detox challenge. Incorporate ways to keep a positive outlook over the long haul.

5.2.3 Long haul Way of life Changes

Feature how the Sweet Opportunity challenge goes about as an impetus for long haul way of life changes. Grandstand accounts of perusers who kept on pursuing educated and quality food decisions past the underlying 3 weeks, stressing that the test fills in as an establishment for practical prosperity.

Urge peruses to share their own examples of overcoming adversity and tributes inside your local area, cultivating a steady climate where people can move and propel one another. Counting a blend of both individual stories and master bits of knowledge will give a balanced viewpoint on the groundbreaking force of embracing a sugar-cognizant way of life.

FAQs and Investigating

6.1 Normal Difficulties Looked During the Test

6.1.1 Sugar Withdrawal Side effects

Address normal side effects experienced during the underlying stage, like cerebral pains, exhaustion, and emotional episodes. Reassure readers that withdrawal symptoms are temporary and a sign that the body is adjusting to a lower sugar intake by providing practical tips for managing them.

6.1.2 Prevalent difficulties and Allurements

Recognize the difficulties of exploring social circumstances where sweet food varieties are pervasive. Offer techniques for courteously declining treats, bringing sans sugar options in contrast to social affairs, and conveying your wellbeing objectives with loved ones.

6.1.3 Profound Eating Triggers

Examine profound eating as a test and give bits of knowledge into perceiving close to home triggers. Share care strategies and elective survival techniques that perusers can use to address profound eating without turning to sweet solace food varieties.

6.2 Master Ways to defeat Snags

6.2.1 Master Counsel on Overseeing Desires

Remember tips from nutritionists or wellbeing experts for how to really oversee and conquer desires. This could include dietary guidance, social methodologies, or care procedures to assist perusers with remaining focused.

6.2.2 Structure an Emotionally supportive network

Underline the significance of an emotionally supportive network during the sugar detox venture. Give master exhortation on building an organization of companions, family, or individual challengers who can offer consolation, share encounters, and give responsibility.

6.2.3 Changing the Test to Individual Necessities

Perceive that everybody's process is exceptional. Offer master guidance on how peruses can fit the sugar detox challenge to accommodate their singular inclinations, dietary requirements, and way of life, guaranteeing a more customized and supportable methodology.

Urge peruses to investigate these FAQs and investigating tips to proactively address difficulties that might emerge during the 3-week challenge. Giving master exhortation adds validity and direction, assisting peruses with exploring likely obstacles with certainty and achievement.

Post-Challenge Support

7.1 Slow renewed introduction of Food varieties

7.1.1 Sluggish and Efficient Methodology

Guide peruses on the most proficient method to once again introduce specific food varieties progressively. Underscore the significance of seeing how their bodies answer different nutrition classes and being aware of any progressions in energy levels, mind-set, or processing.

7.1.2 Distinguishing Trigger Food varieties

Assist peruses with perceiving potential trigger food varieties that might prompt desires or undesirable responses. Empower keeping a renewed introduction diary to follow reactions to various food varieties, considering informed choices about what to remember for their continuous eating regimen.

7.2 Consolidating Treats With some restraint

7.2.1 Careful Guilty pleasure

Talk about the idea of careful extravagance, where treats are appreciated deliberately and with some restraint. Provide advice on how to avoid overindulging in sweets and encourage readers to indulge occasionally without guilt.

7.2.2 Solid Other options

Propose better choices for sweet treats, for example, custom made pastries with regular sugars or natural product based choices. Provide recipes and concepts that are in line with incorporating treats into a regular eating plan in a way that is both balanced and mindful.

7.3 Developing a Long-Term Health Plan 7.3.1 Establishing Long-Term Goals Aid readers in establishing long-term health objectives that are both attainable and sustainable. Energize a comprehensive methodology that thinks about active work, hydration, and generally speaking prosperity, not simply dietary decisions.

7.3.2 Customary Wellbeing Registrations

Advocate for customary self-appraisal and registrations to assess headway and make important changes. Urge perusers to stand by listening to their bodies, adjust their arrangements depending on the situation, and celebrate progressing triumphs in keeping a fair and sound way of life.

7.3.3 Looking for Proficient Direction

Feature the significance of talking with medical services experts, nutritionists, or dietitians for customized exhortation. Give assets and tips on finding neighborhood or online experts who can offer direction in view of individual wellbeing needs and objectives.

Integrate useful hints, examples of overcoming adversity from the individuals who effectively kept a sugar-cognizant way of life post-challenge, and updates that the excursion is progressing. The objective is to engage peruses to keep settling on informed decisions for their wellbeing while at the same time partaking in an economical and offset relationship with food.

End

8.1 Considering Your Sweet Opportunity Excursion

8.1.1 Recognizing Accomplishments

Pause for a minute for self-reflection and commend the accomplishments made during the 3-week Sweet Opportunity challenge. Urge per users to perceive the advancement they've achieved, both of all shapes and sizes, and offer thanks for the positive changes experienced.

8.1.2 Illustrations Learned

Ponder the examples advanced all through the excursion. Discuss the new information regarding cravings for sugar and healthier alternatives. Welcome peruses to consider how these examples can be applied to their continuous relationship with food.

8.2 Pushing Ahead with a Better Relationship with Sugar

8.2.1 Embracing a Way of life Shift

Urge peruses to see the Sweet Opportunity challenge as an impetus for a way of life shift as opposed to a momentary fix.

Accentuate the significance of supporting the positive propensities created during the test and incorporating them into their day to day existences.

8.2.2 Flexibility and Balance In order to maintain a healthier relationship with sugar, discuss the idea of flexibility and balance. Remind peruses that periodic extravagances are an ordinary piece of life and that the key is to move toward them carefully, keeping generally wellbeing and prosperity in center.

8.2.3 Associating with the Local area

Urge peruses to remain associated with the local area shaped during the test. Share ways of keeping on supporting and propelling one another, whether through web-based entertainment gatherings, standard registrations, or taking part in continuous difficulties.

8.2.4 Defining Future Wellbeing Objectives

Motivate peruses to lay out new wellbeing objectives in light of their singular requirements and goals. Give direction on making a guide for future wellbeing and prosperity, underscoring the significance of progressing personal development.

In the determination, convey a feeling of achievement and strengthening. Remind readers that their Sweet Freedom journey is a stepping stone toward a healthier and more balanced lifestyle rather than a destination. Encourage them to embrace the never-ending process of learning, adjusting, and savoring a life of sweet freedom.

<u>Please leave a review and appreciate</u>